A Yoga Guide for Kids

Start Yoga Young. Benefit for a lifetime.

Introducing Your Instructor Yog-Hee™

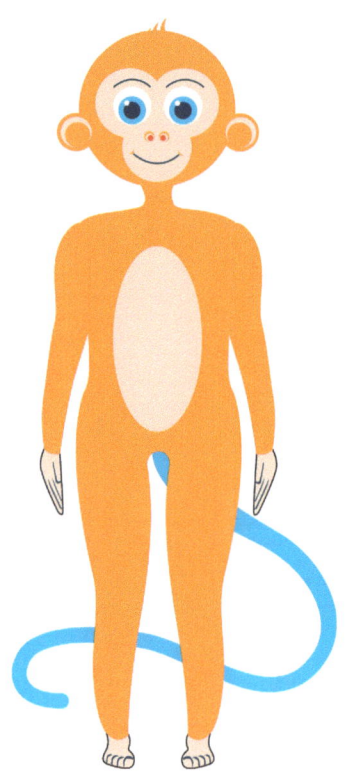

Author: Vasudha Badri-Paul

Illustrations: Rahul Verma

Creative Director: Nirand Salian

Editor: Jaya Hoy

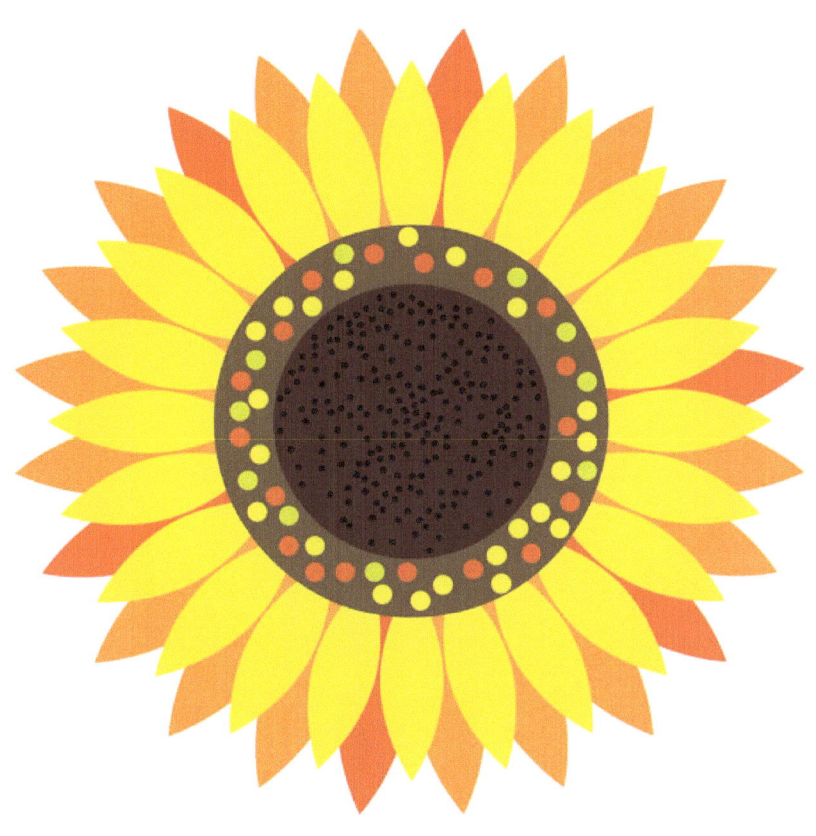

Dedicated to all the kids in the world.

My family. My friends

Acknowledgment:

To all the yoga teachers who have contributed to my journey so far. I thank you all. A very special thanks to my first guru in India, Mrs. Rajeswari Raman. She was my first guide and started me on my path when I was 10 years old. I treasure her yoga book "Hatha Yoga for All" and remember her very fondly.

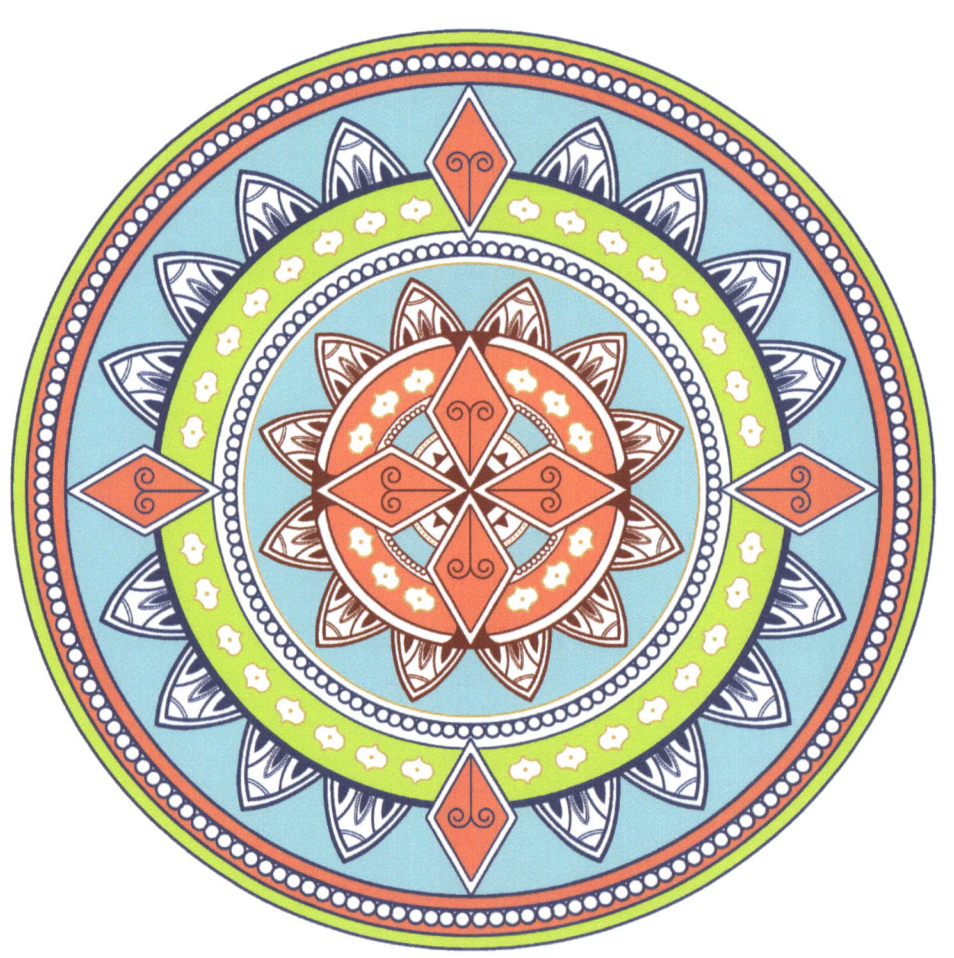

When You Practice Yoga Once a Week, You Change Your Mind

When You Practice Yoga Once a Week, You Change Your Body

When You Practice Yoga Every Day, It Will Change Your Life

-Unknown

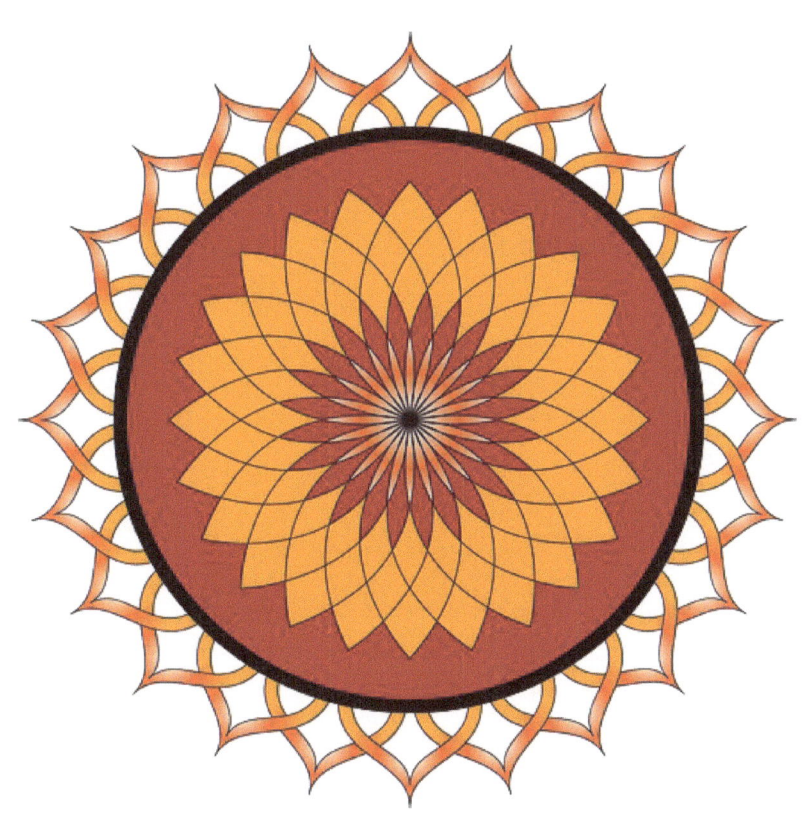

Introduction

Yoga is a complete science of living that has origins in ancient India. Yoga balances the mind, body, and spirit and brings about deep harmony in one's life. Children are starting their life journey and can benefit deeply from the practice of yoga, however simple. The practices in this book can serve as the building blocks for a lifetime of yoga that will help them in all aspects of life. The physical asanas, the meditation practice, and the breathing practice will be their companion in countless ways, making them happier, healthier human beings with a deeper reserve of inner strength. Yoga will give them the tools to face the inevitable obstacles in life and overcome them with a peaceful approach.

The book is a basic recipe of yoga poses, breathing, and meditation for kids. The food section is added as good nutrition is essential for health, especially for a growing body.

A Note About Practice:

1. Practice should be at the same time every day (as far as possible). Regularity is important
2. A yoga mat or a regular mat should be used for practice
3. An adult can start the practice along with the child
4. The practice should be done at least half an hour after light eating. After a heavy meal, wait at least 2 hours
5. All asanas do not have to be done at every sitting. One can choose asanas for each practice session, but they should be combined with one breathing exercise and meditation as an ending to realize the full benefits of the practice
6. You can split the practice into 10-15 minutes in the morning and 10-15 minutes in the evening

Table of Contents

Chapter 1

Yoga Asanas (Exercises)

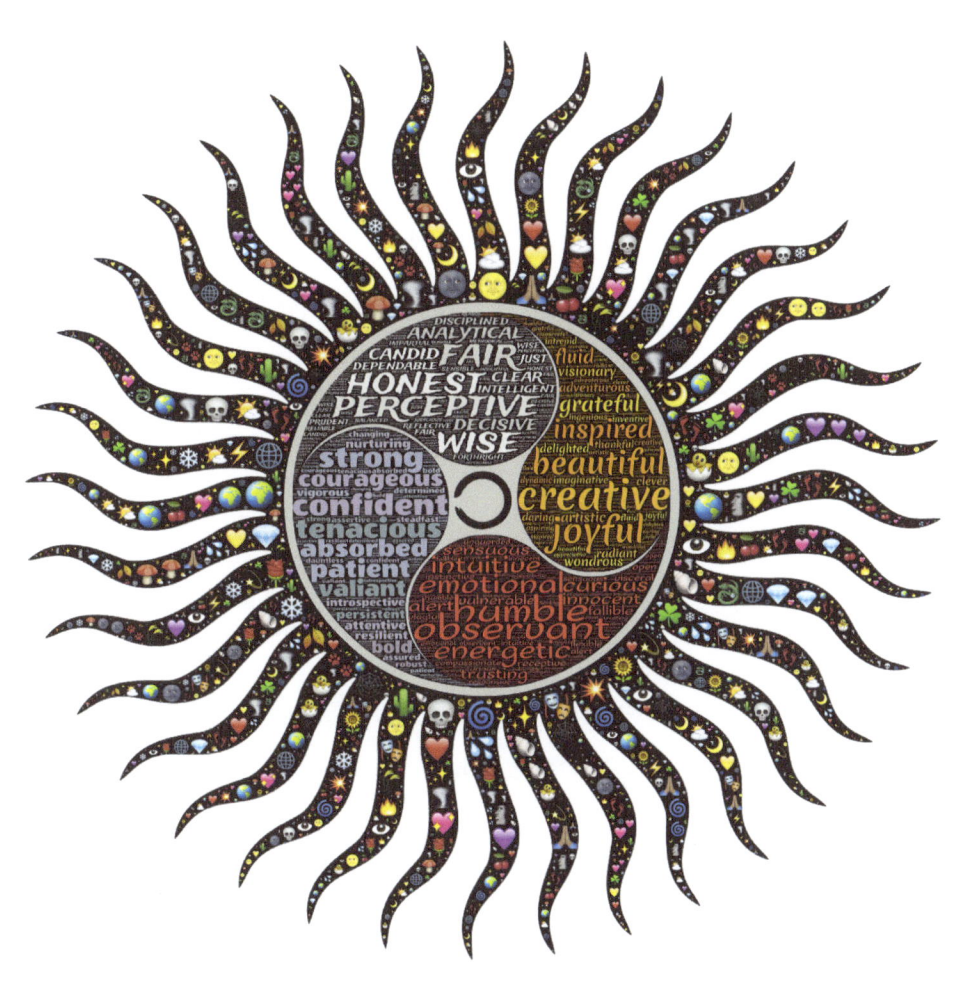

1. *Sunrise-Sunset Asana*
   Key Benefits: warm-up, stretches the entire body

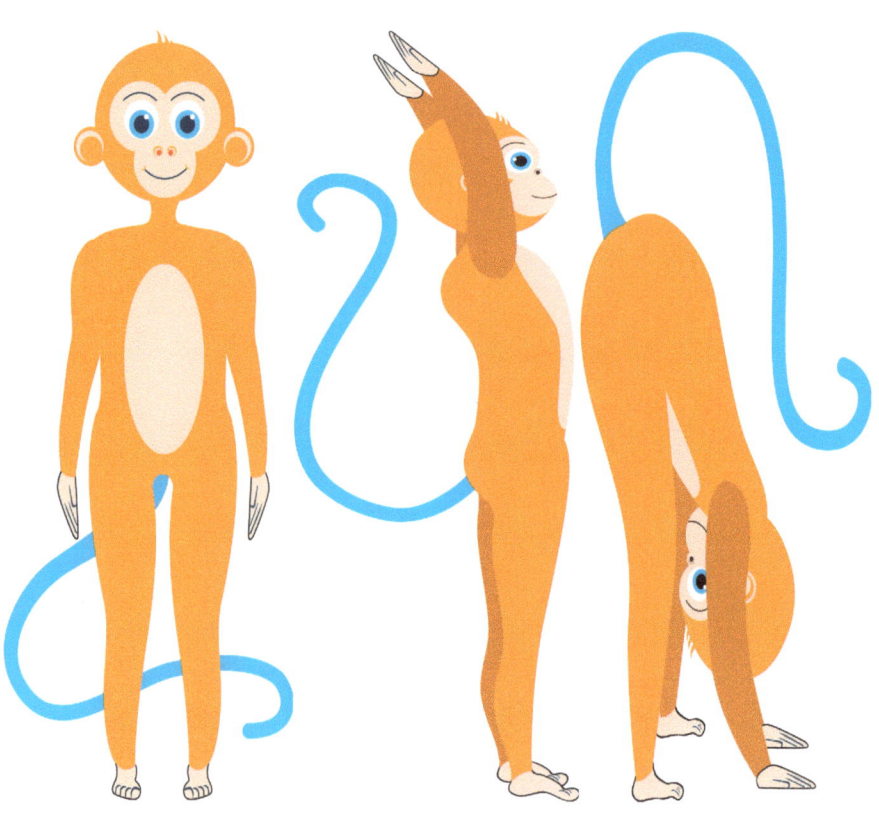

1. Stand with the feet shoulder-width apart, hands at the side
2. Breathing in, slowly raise both hands over the head, stretching with palms facing outwards
3. Hold the pose for a slow count of 3
4. Breathing out, slowly bring the hands to the floor until the palms are close to or flat on the floor.
5. Hold the pose for a slow count of 6
6. Breathing in, come back to the pose with hands at the side
7. Pause for a slow count of 3 and repeat the asana 2 more times

2. Tree Asana

Key Benefits: Balance, endurance, and alertness

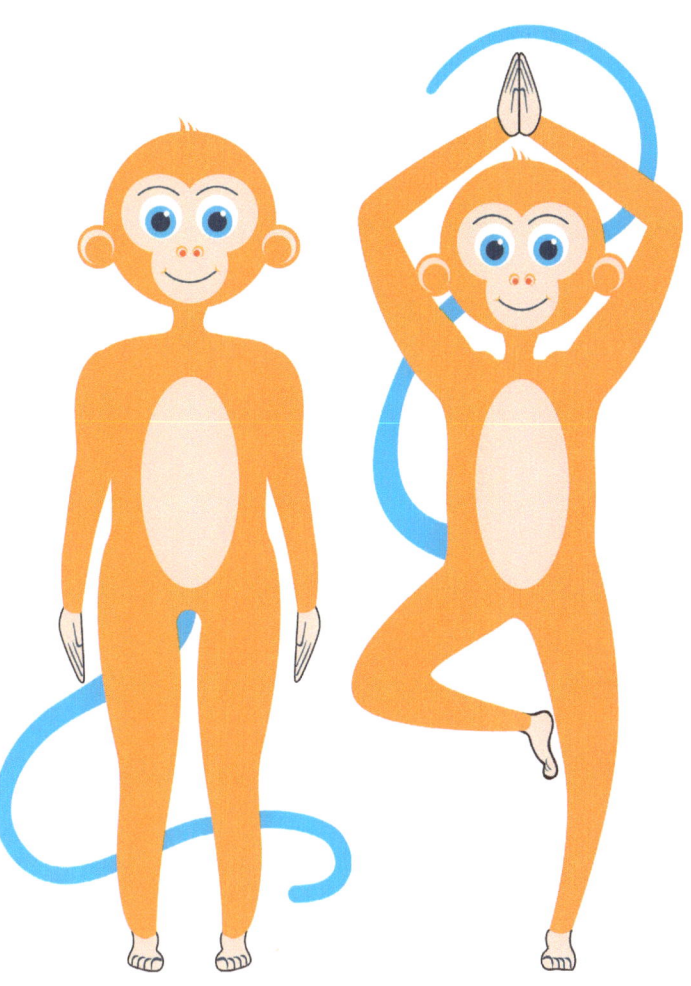

1. *Stand with feet together, hands at the side*

2. *Breathe in and raise right leg. Bring it to rest on the inner right thigh*

3. *Move hands upwards to prayer pose (if you feel unsteady, release and come back to standing pose)*

4. *Hold for the slow count of 6, breathing normally*

5. *Take a deep breath and bring the leg down while breathing out and releasing the hands to the sides*

6. *Repeat with the left leg*

7. *Repeat asana 2 more times*

3. Bridge Asana
Key Benefits: Balance, endurance, and alertness

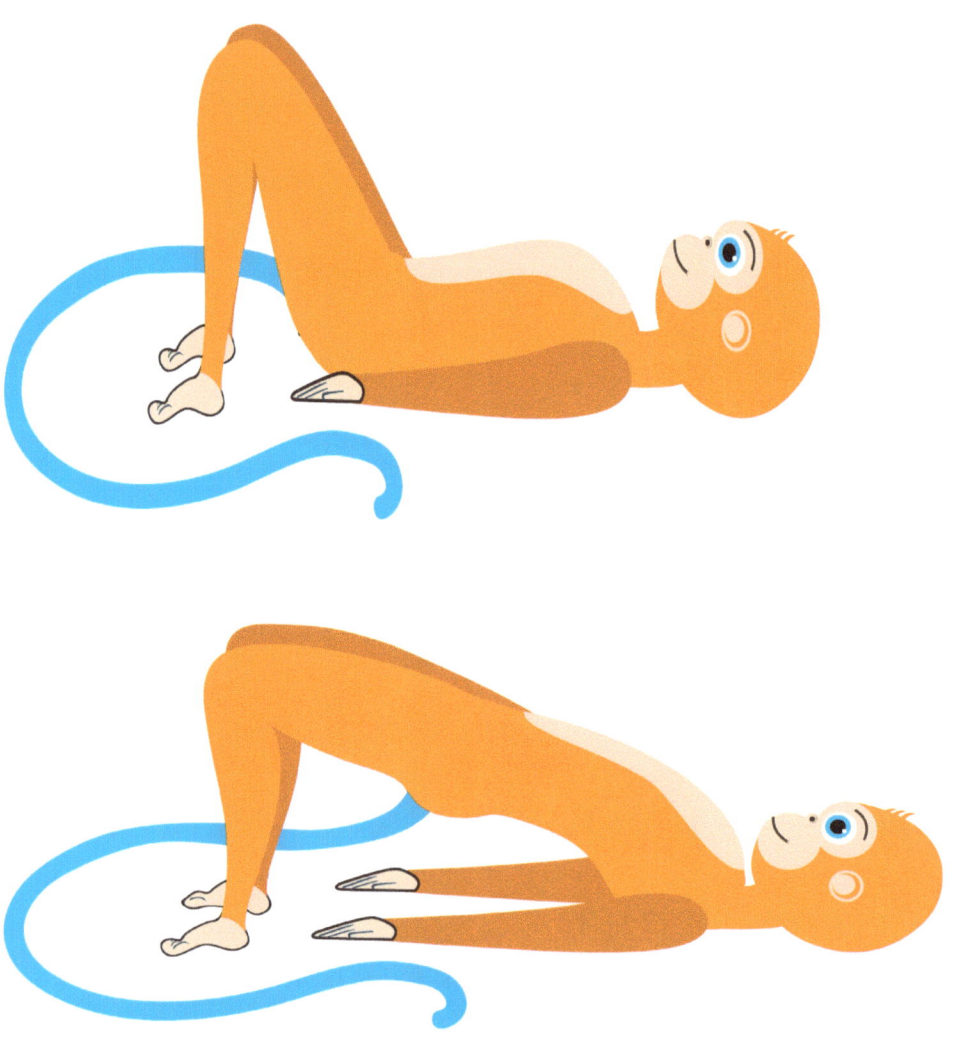

1. Lie down with back on floor, palms down, hips a few inches apart. Bend legs

2. Breathing in, gently raise your hips off the floor to form a bridge

3. Hold for a slow count of 6

4. Breath in and breathe out as you release your hips back to the floor

5. Pause for a slow count of 6

6. Repeat 4 more times

4. Snake Asana
Key Benefits: Balance, endurance, and alertness

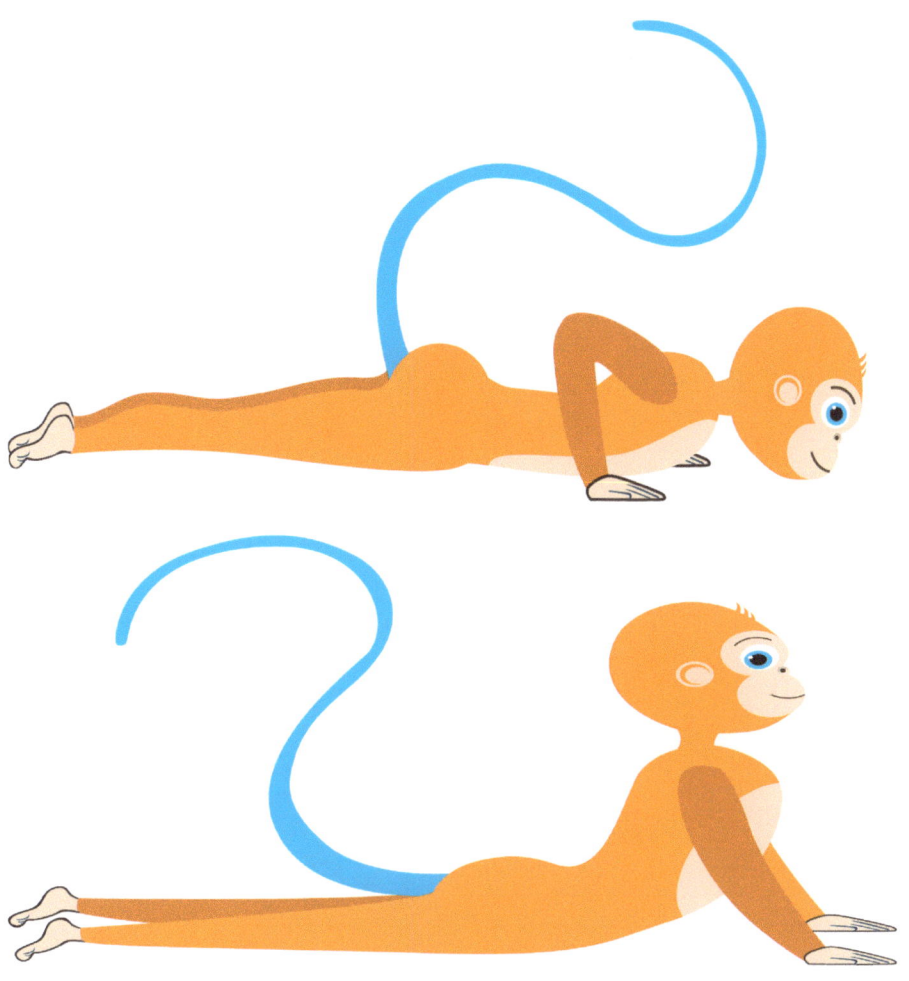

1. *Lie on stomach, forearms on ground, elbows beneath shoulders and palms pressed to the ground. Chin on ground as shown in diagram above.*
2. *Keeping hips on the ground, breathe in and gently lift head and chest until hands are straight. Make sure shoulder is back in final position so that the chest opens up.*
3. *Hold and breathe normally for a slow count of 5*
4. *Take a deep breath and as you breathe out, bring your upper body back to the ground*
5. *Pause for 6 slow breaths*
6. *Repeat 4 more times*

5. Cow-Cat Asana
Key Benefits: Balance, endurance, and
alertness

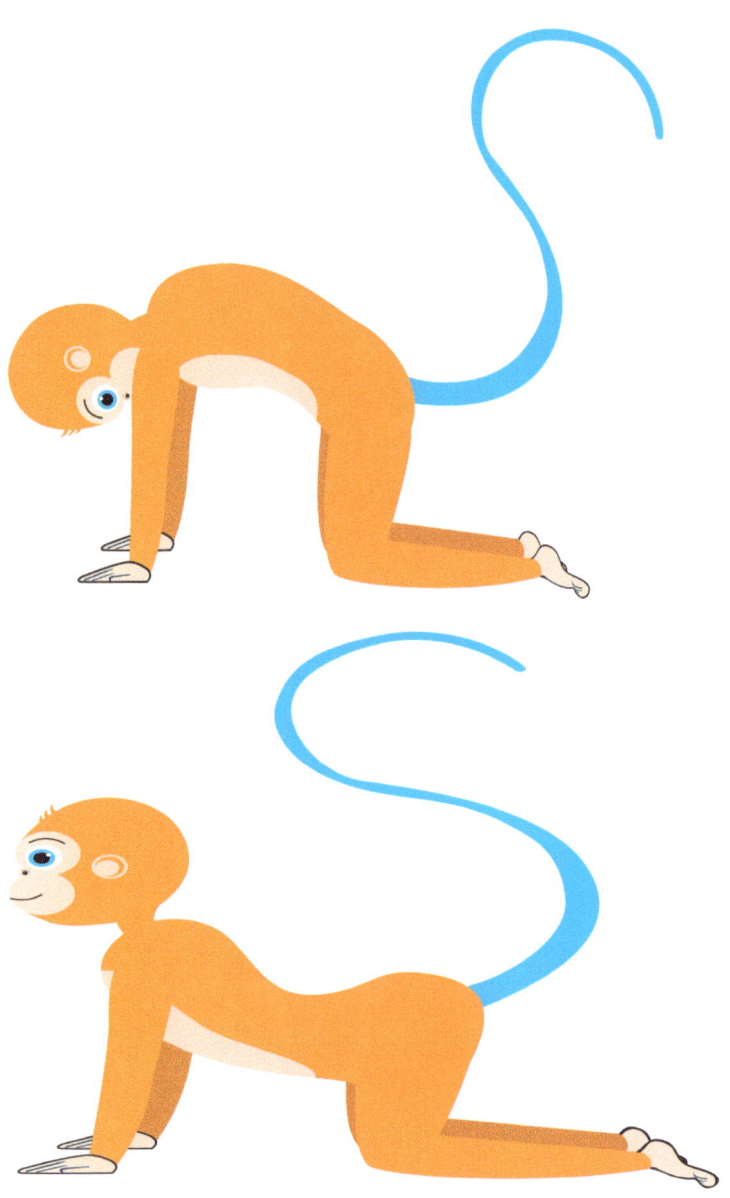

1. Get onto all fours

2. Breathing in, slowly raise head up and arch lower back down (cat)

3. Hold for a slow count of 3

4. Breathing out, slowly drop your head down and arch back upwards (cow)

5. Hold for a slow count of 3

6. Repeat cat and cow pose 4 more times. Remember to do movements slowly

6. Downward Monkey
Key Benefits: Energizes, builds upper body strength

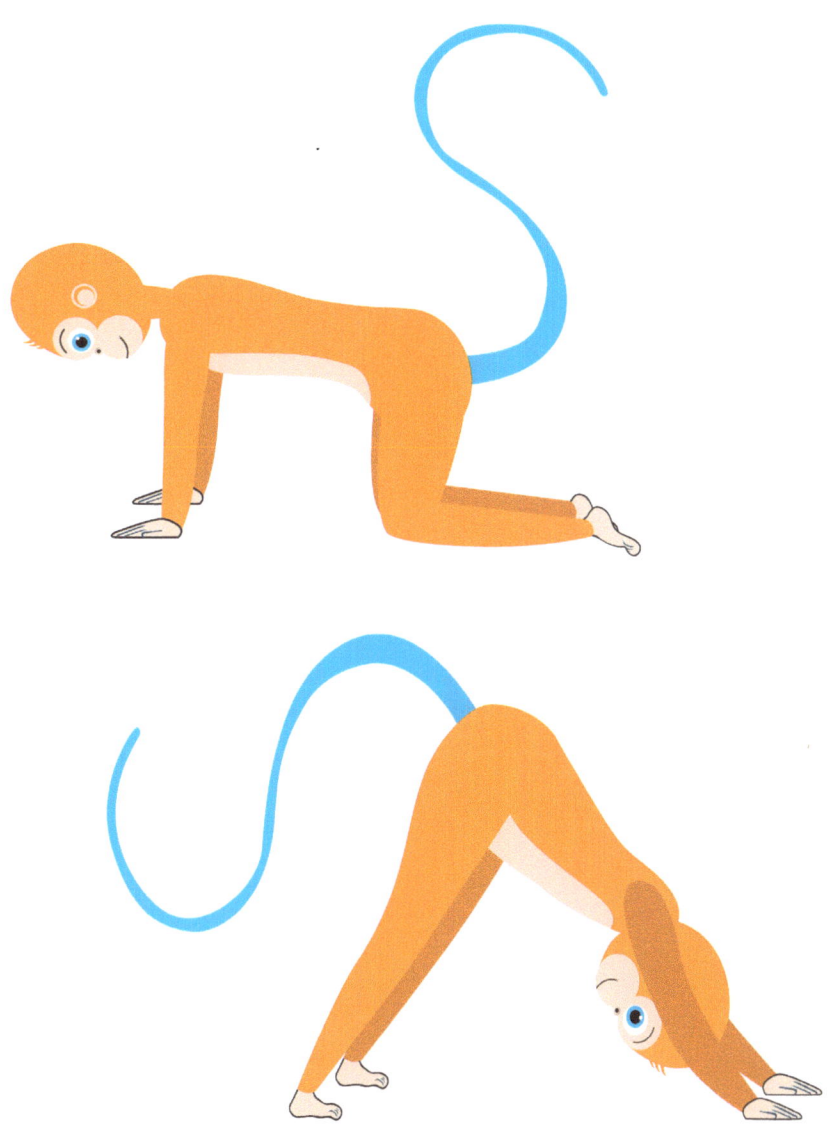

1. *Get down on all fours*
2. *Slowly raise your hips until your feet are straightened and your head is between your hands*
3. *Stay in the position for a slow count of 6*
4. *Come back to all fours*
5. *Pause for a slow count of 6*
6. *Repeat asana 4 more times*

7. Plank Asana
Key Benefits: Strengthens core

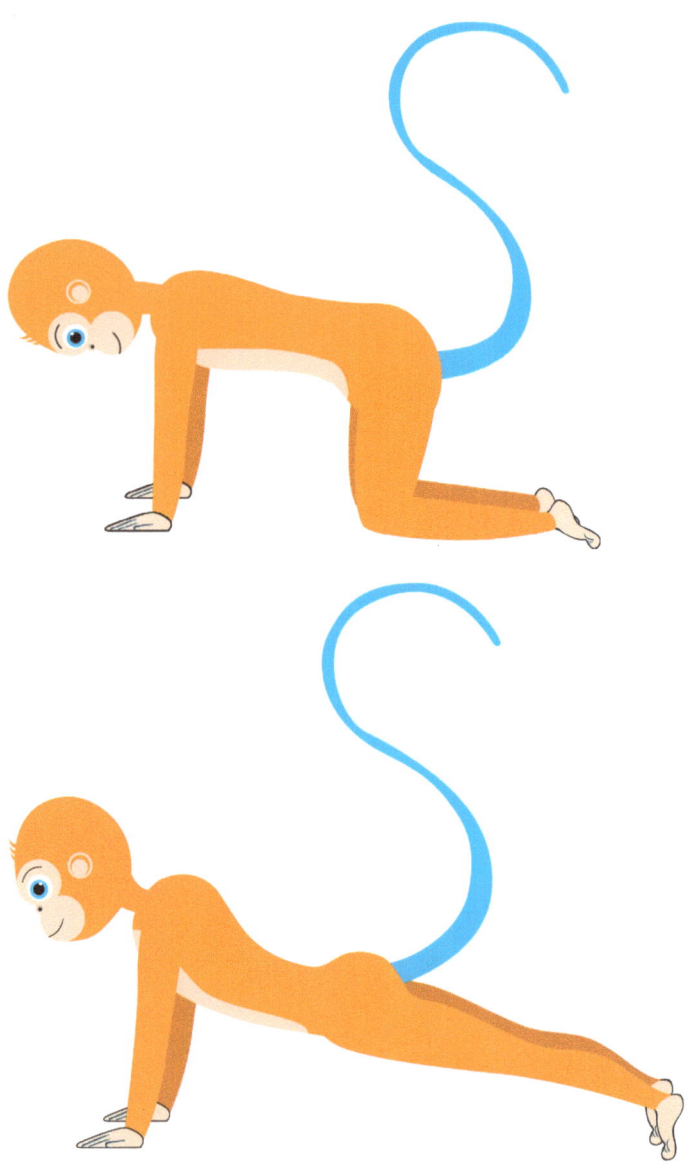

1. *Get down on all fours*

2. *Move your right and then left foot back*

3. *Pretend to be an alligator floating in the water*

4. *Hold the position for 25-30 seconds, breathing normally*

5. *Breathe in and come back to all fours*

6. *Repeat 1 more time*

8. Garland Asana

Key Benefits: Strengthens core and hips, calms

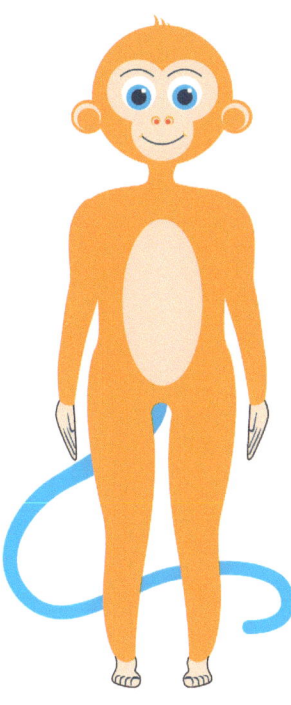

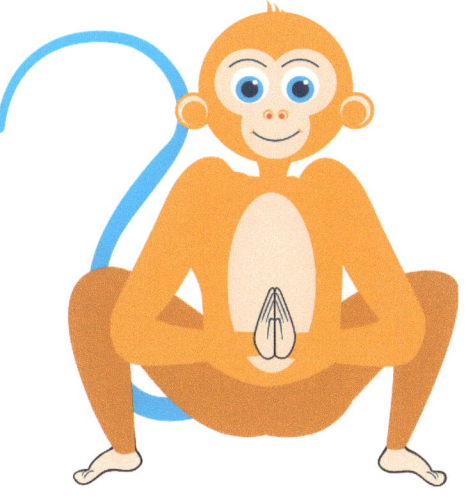

1. *Stand with palms facing out and away from body, legs shoulder-width apart*
2. *Take a deep breath. While breathing out, move your body down into a squat*
3. *Bring hands to prayer pose*
4. *Breathe normally to a slow count of 10*
5. *Breathing out, come back to standing position*
6. *Repeat asana 4 times*

9. Boat Asana

Key Benefits: Strengthens hip, core, spine

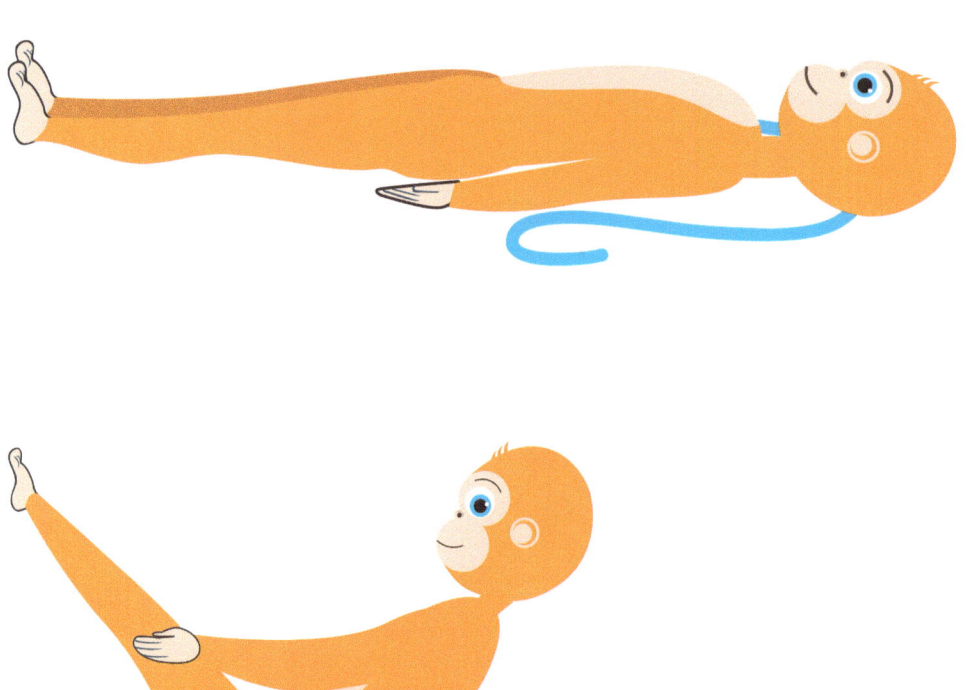

1. *Lie down on your back with your legs in front of you*
2. *Take a deep breath and breathing out, lift your legs off the floor until you are balancing on your hips. Bring your hands forward*
3. *Hold for a slow count of 6*
4. *Breath out as you lower your body to the ground*
5. *Repeat 4 more times*

10. Airplane Asana
Key Benefits: Balance, strengthens arms, shoulders, hips

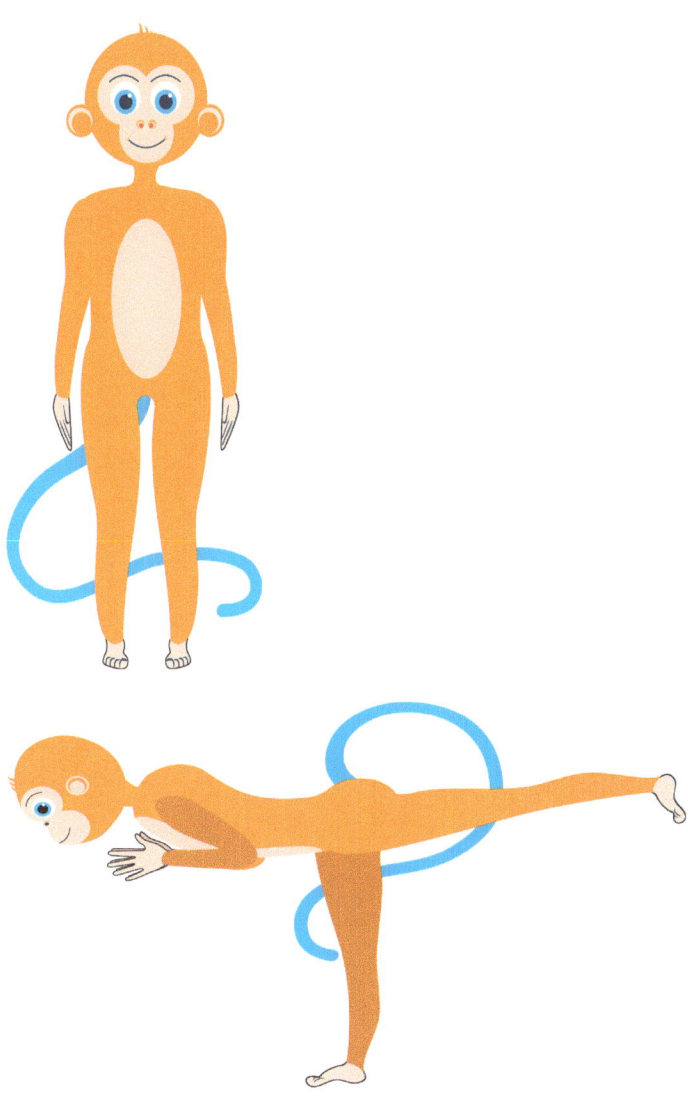

1. *Stand with legs together. Hands at side.*

2. *Breathing in deeply, slowly bend your body forward while raising your right leg*

3. *Place palms together. Hold for a slow count of 6*

4. *Breathe out, release palms and slowly come back to the starting position and relax for a slow count of 6*

5. *Repeat with left leg*

6. *Repeat the series 3 more times*

11. Butterfly Asana
Key Benefits: Opens and stretches hips

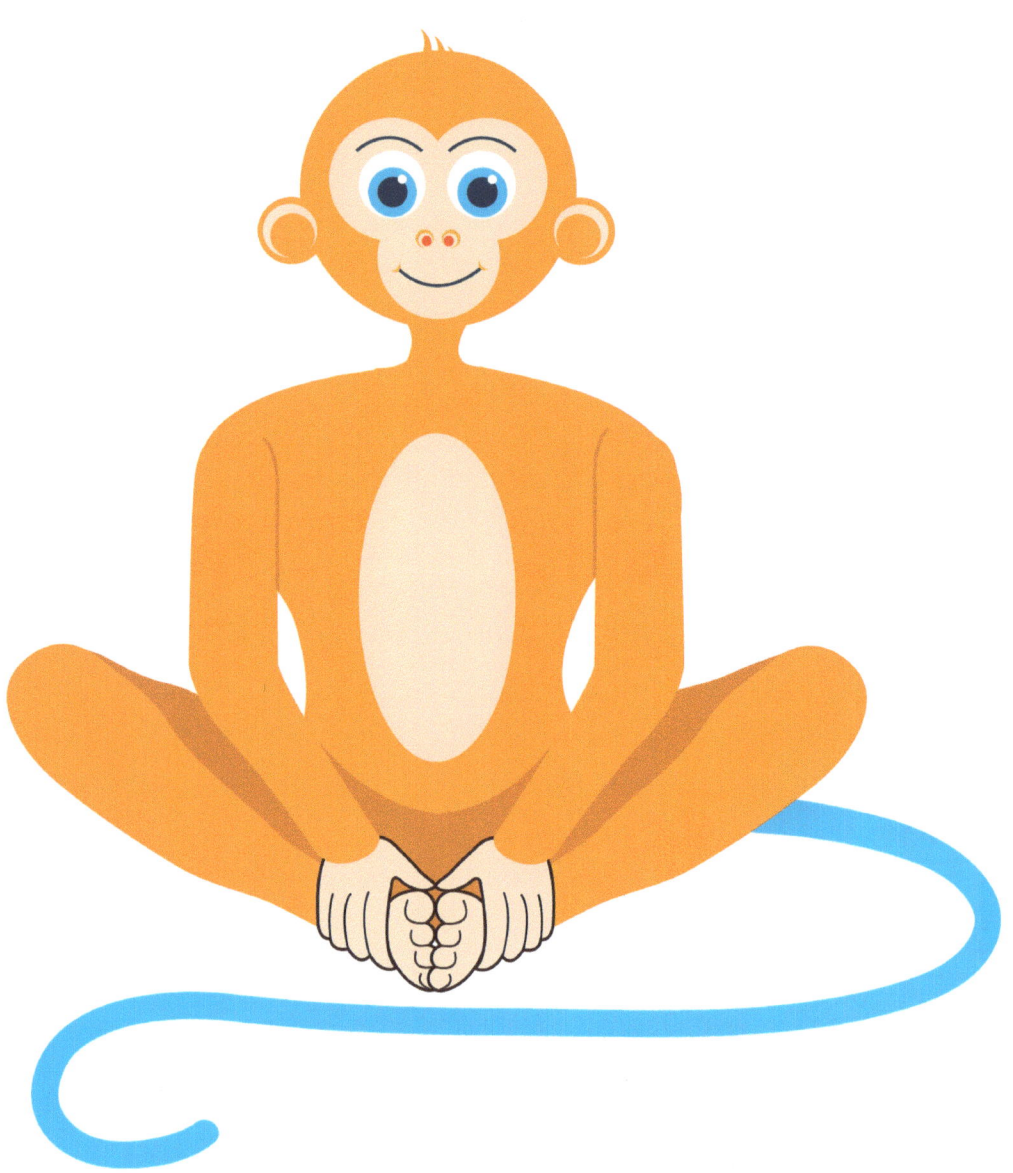

- Sit up tall. Bring the soles of your feet together
- Flap the legs like a butterfly, making slow up and down movements.
- Do this for a slow count of 10-15
- Pause for a count of 12
- Repeat 2 more times

12. Child Asana

Key Benefits: Calms body, mind. Relaxes neck, shoulders

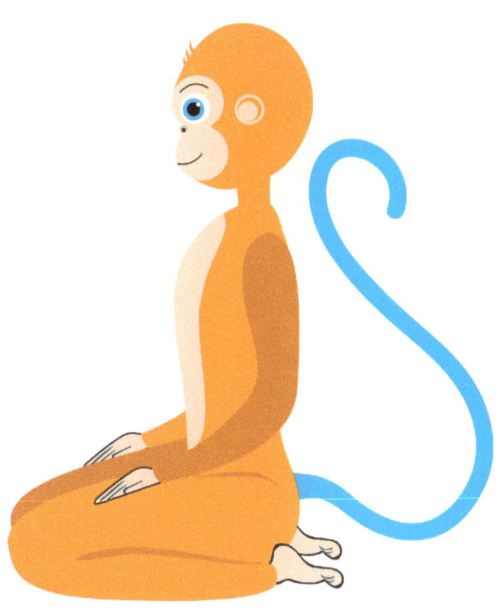

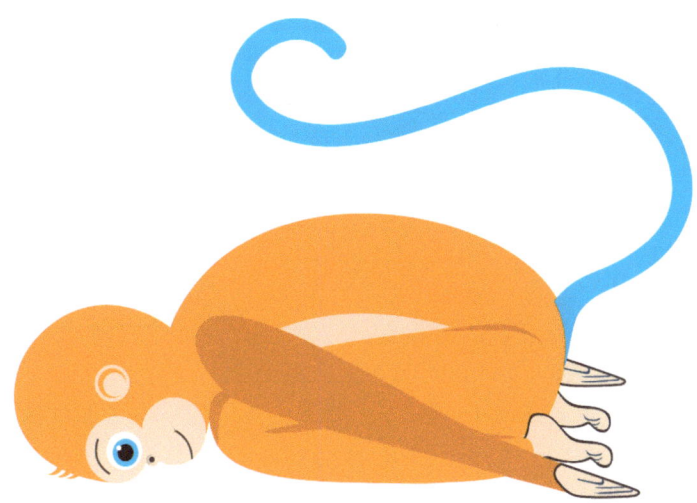

1. Sit with legs under hips
2. Take a deep breath. Slowly breathe out and move your body downwards until your forehead touches the floor
3. Bring your arms back alongside your thighs with the palms facing upwards
4. Stay for 1 minute and focus on your inhalations and exhalations
5. Sit up and get ready for breathing pose

Chapter 2
Breathing

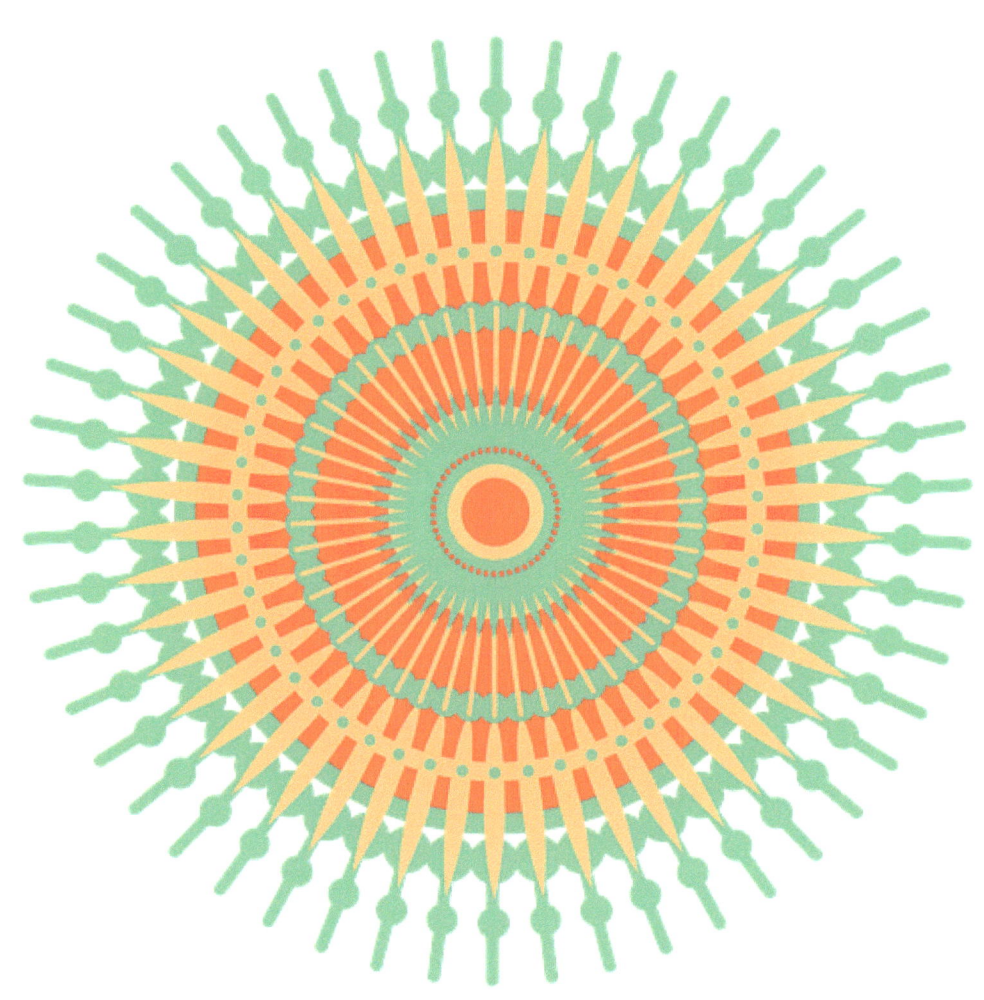

13. Breathing like a Bee

Key Benefits: Improves memory and concentration, relieves anxiety

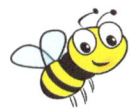

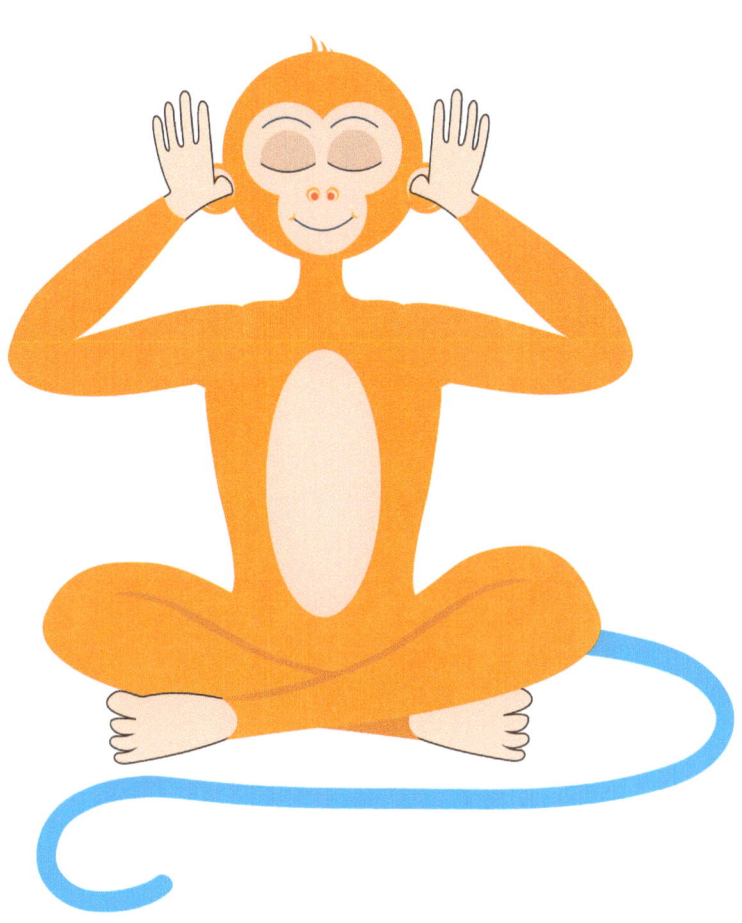

1. Sit with legs comfortably crossed
2. Watch your breath go in and out for a slow count of 5
3. Take a deep breath
4. Gently place your thumbs in your ears and hum like a bee (hmmmmmm) as you breathe out. Pause.
5. Remove your thumbs and bring hands down to your lap
6. Relax for a few seconds while watching your breath
7. Repeat 3 more times

Chapter 3
Meditation

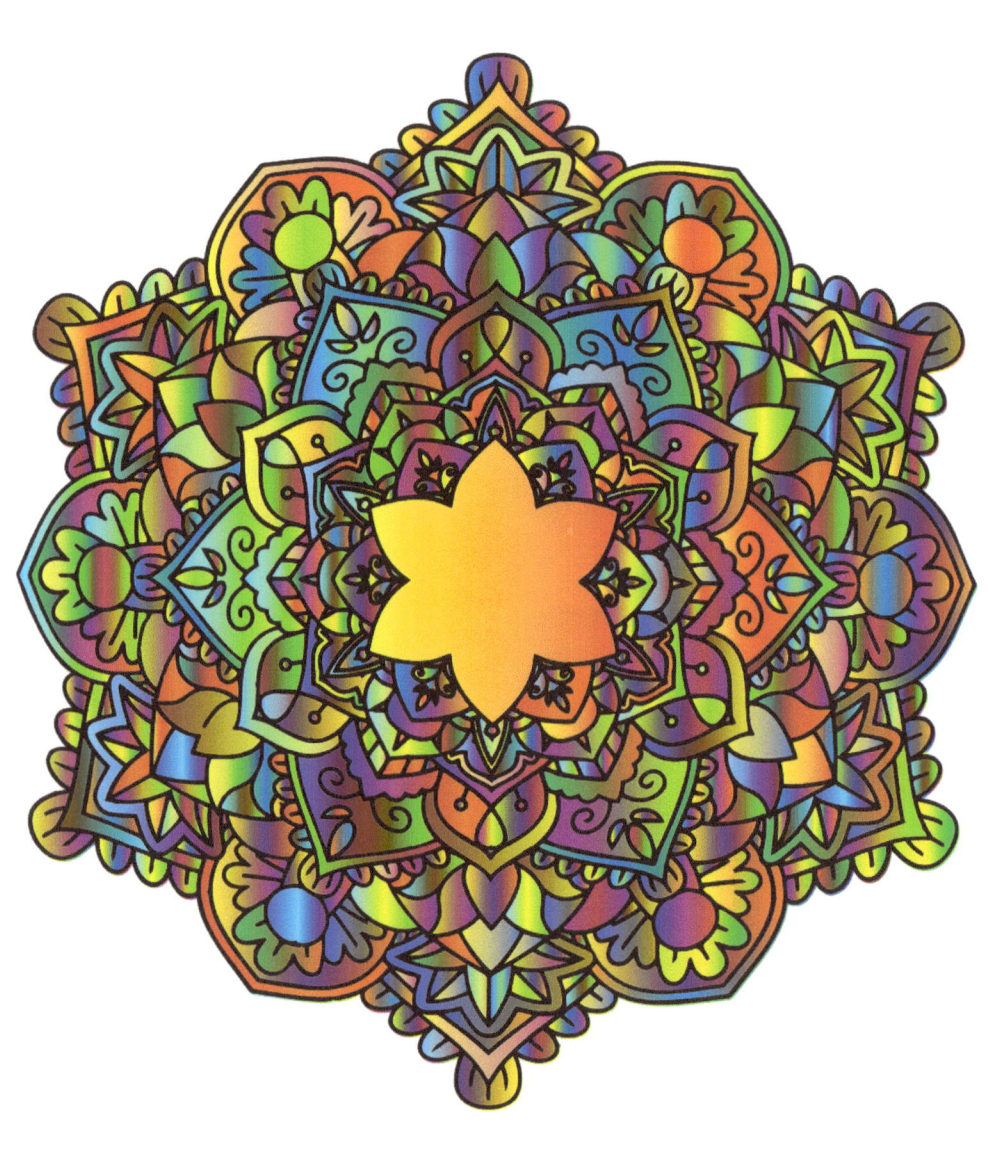

14. Balloon Meditation
Key Benefits: Calms mind and body

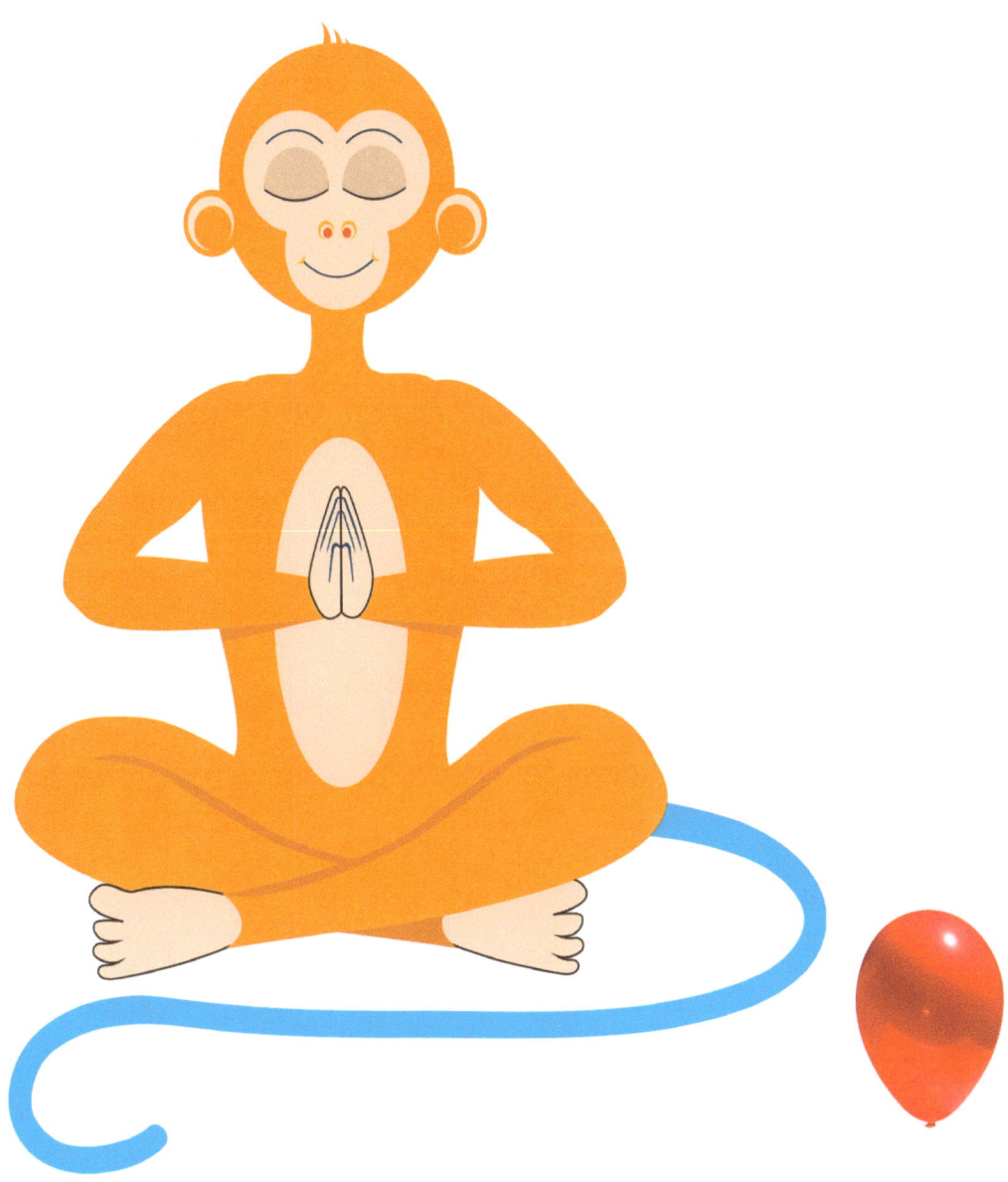

1. Sit down cross-legged and close your eyes

2. Take 1 deep inhalation to a slow count of 4 and release

3. Inhale and fill your belly with as much air as possible extending it as if you were blowing a balloon

4. Exhale slowly with a "hisssss" and pretend that the balloon is releasing air. Relax your body with the exhalation. Pause

5. Repeat 3-5 times

15. Watching the breath
Key Benefits: Calms mind and body

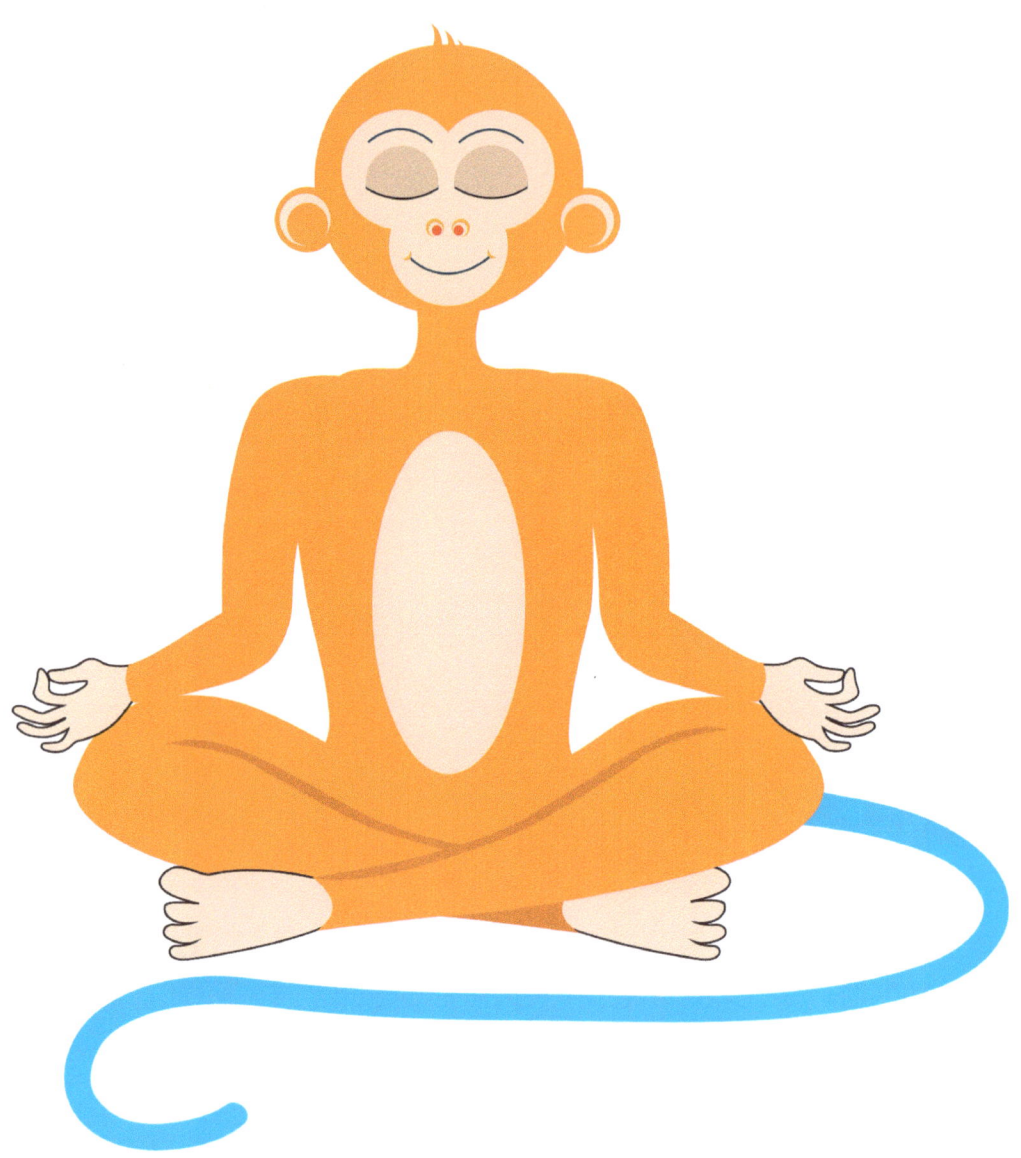

1. Sit cross-legged. Inhale slowly for a count of 5, counting on your fingers. Pause for 2 counts

2. Exhale slowly for 5 counts, counting on fingers

3. Feel the air come in and out of your nose as you breathe in and out

4. Repeat 3 more times.

5. Sit still and watch your breath for 30 seconds to 1 minute at the end

Chapter 4
Food for Health

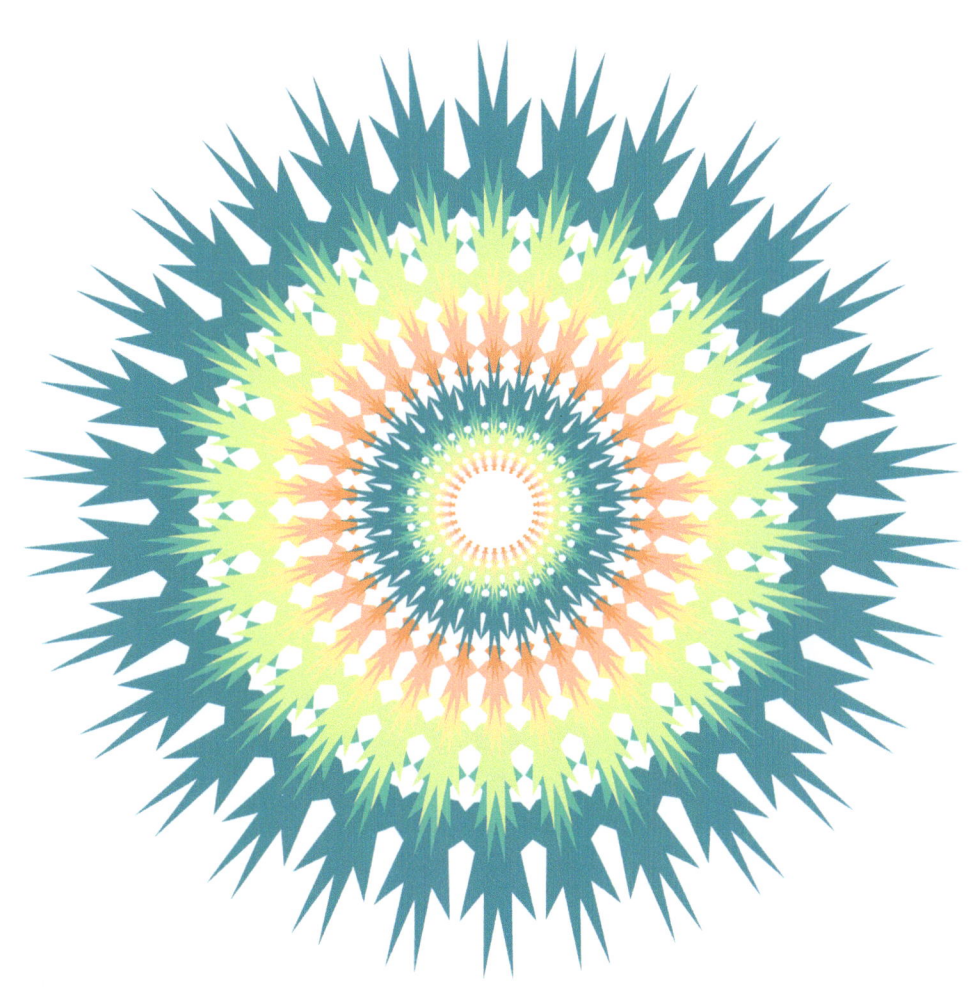

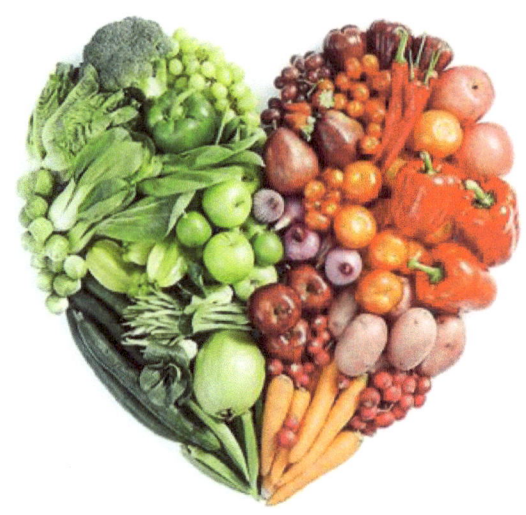

Food is essential for a healthy body and it is always good to start good habits young. Like anything else, you can help children develop good eating habits.

You can start by including leafy greens and other vegetables in their diet. Leafy greens are rich in iron and fiber. Make meals more appealing by using colorful fruits, nuts, and whole grains. Prepare salads and make them a part of a daily diet. By giving the child fruits and vegetables regularly, it will soon become a habit.

Make it a practice to practice what you preach – seeing you eat a salad or fresh fruit with relish, kids will find eating healthy foods more pleasant and enjoyable. Avoid or minimize giving junk food and processed food to children. Most processed food contains harmful additives, preservatives, extra sodium, and fat. Help kids become aware of the harmful effects of junk food and the benefits of nutritious food. This is one of the good habits that you should instill in your kids for them to enjoy the benefits of a healthier body.

Final words*:*

It is your responsibility as a parent to guide your kids in establishing a healthy lifestyle. The practice of yoga can contribute deeply to the growth of your child in many ways: physical, mental, and emotional. Start the practice slowly and make it enjoyable. They will reap more than they sow if they include a steady yoga practice in their life.

Yoga Thoughts:

I have an attitude of gratitude

I respect all living beings and nature

I am willing to serve the community

I am strong. I believe in myself. I can overcome all obstacles

I am happy

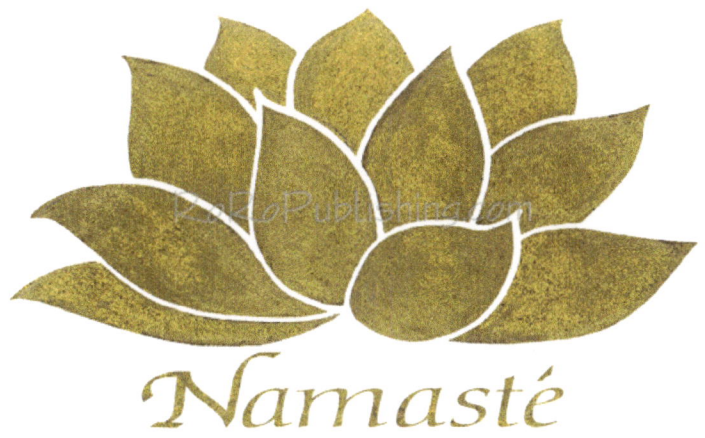

Namasté

About the Author:

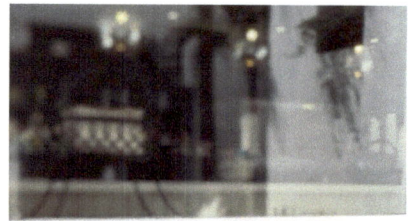

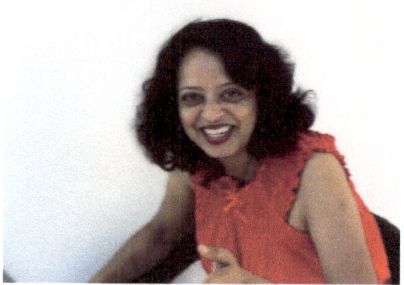

Vasudha Badri-Paul teaches children yoga as an after-school activity in the school district in California. She also has classes for women and organizes yoga camps in the summer where kids are taught yoga and some basic healthy cooking skills. Her website is www.yogachimps.com. She learnt yoga as a child in India and truly believes in teaching yoga at a young age to make it a lifelong companion.

Vasudha lives in the Bay Area, California, and works in the technology industry. Besides yoga, she loves hiking, reading, and creative writing.